I0696992

Healthy Hearts Cookbook

Nutritious and Flavorful Recipes for Heart Disease Prevention

Tony Duncan

All rights reserved. No part of this publication may be reproduced, distributed, or transmitted in any form or by any means, including photocopying, recording, or other electronic or mechanical methods, without the prior written permission of the publisher, except in the case of brief quotations embodied in critical reviews and certain other noncommercial uses permitted by copyright law.

Copyright © Tony Duncan, 2023.

Content

Chapter 1: Heart-Healthy Breakfast Ideas

Berry Oatmeal Delight:

This recipe is a heart-healthy breakfast option that provides a good source of fiber and antioxidants. Fiber helps to lower cholesterol levels, while antioxidants support heart health by reducing inflammation and protecting against oxidative stress.

Ingredients:

- 1 cup rolled oats: Oats are rich in soluble fiber, which can help lower cholesterol levels.
- 2 cups of water or milk (such as almond milk): Choose low-fat milk or unsweetened almond milk to reduce saturated fat intake.
- 1 cup mixed berries (such as strawberries, blueberries, raspberries): Berries are packed with antioxidants, vitamins, and minerals that benefit heart health.

- 1 tablespoon honey or maple syrup (optional): Use sparingly, if desired, as a natural sweetener.
- 1 tablespoon chia seeds (optional): Chia seeds are a great source of omega-3 fatty acids, fiber, and antioxidants.
- A sprinkle of cinnamon: Cinnamon has been linked to improved heart health by helping to regulate blood sugar and cholesterol levels.

Instructions:

1. Combine rolled oats and water or milk in a saucepan and bring to a boil.
2. Reduce heat and simmer for about 5 minutes until the oats reach desired consistency, stirring occasionally.
3. Remove from heat and add mixed berries, honey or maple syrup (if desired), chia seeds, and cinnamon. Mix well.
4. Allow the mixture to sit for a few minutes to allow the berries to soften.
5. Serve warm and enjoy a heart-healthy and satisfying breakfast.

Avocado Toast with Poached Egg:

This recipe provides heart-healthy fats from avocado and protein from eggs. Avocado is a great source of monounsaturated fats that can help lower LDL (bad) cholesterol levels.

Ingredients:

- 2 slices of whole wheat bread: Whole wheat bread is higher in fiber and nutrients compared to refined white bread.
- 1 ripe avocado: Avocado provides heart-healthy monounsaturated fats, fiber, and vitamins.
- Juice of half a lemon: Lemon juice adds flavor and provides vitamin C.
- Salt and pepper to taste: Use in moderation to control sodium intake.
- 2 large eggs, poached: Eggs are a good source of protein and essential nutrients.
- Optional toppings: sliced tomatoes, microgreens, or red pepper flakes can add extra flavor and nutrients.

Instructions:

1. Toast whole wheat bread until desired level of crispness.
2. In a small bowl, mash the ripe avocado with lemon juice, salt, and pepper until well combined.
3. Spread the avocado mixture evenly on the toasted bread slices.
4. Place a poached egg on top of each avocado toast.
5. Garnish with optional toppings like sliced tomatoes, microgreens, or red pepper flakes.
6. Sprinkle with a pinch of salt and pepper if desired.
7. Serve immediately and enjoy a heart-healthy and protein-packed breakfast.

Veggie Omelet:

This recipe is a nutritious option packed with vegetables, protein, and essential vitamins and minerals. Vegetables provide fiber, antioxidants, and various nutrients that support heart health.

Ingredients:

- 3 large eggs: Eggs are a good source of protein, vitamins, and minerals.
- 1/4 cup chopped bell peppers (assorted colors): Bell peppers are rich in antioxidants and vitamin C.
- 1/4 cup chopped spinach: Spinach is a nutrient-dense leafy green that provides vitamins, minerals, and antioxidants.
- 1/4 cup diced tomatoes: Tomatoes contain lycopene, an antioxidant associated with heart health.
- 2 tablespoons diced onions: Onions add flavor and contain antioxidants that benefit heart health.
- 1 tablespoon olive oil: Olive oil is a healthy fat that can help reduce LDL (bad) cholesterol levels.
- Salt and pepper to taste: Use in moderation to control sodium intake.
- Optional: shredded low-fat cheese (such as mozzarella or feta) can be added for flavor.

Instructions:

1. In a bowl, whisk the eggs until well beaten. Season with salt and pepper.
2. Heat olive oil in a non-stick skillet over medium heat.
3. Add chopped bell peppers, spinach, tomatoes, and onions to the skillet. Sauté for a few minutes until the vegetables are slightly softened.
4. Pour the beaten eggs over the sautéed vegetables in the skillet.
5. Gently stir the mixture with a spatula to distribute the vegetables evenly.
6. Cook for about 2-3 minutes or until the omelet is mostly set.
7. If desired, sprinkle shredded low-fat cheese over half of the omelet.
8. Fold the other half of the omelet over the cheese side and cook for an additional minute until the cheese melts.
9. Slide the omelet onto a plate and let it cool for a minute before serving.

10. Serve warm and enjoy a nutrient-packed and heart-healthy breakfast.

Greek Yogurt Parfait:

This recipe combines Greek yogurt, fruits, and nuts to create a delicious and heart-healthy breakfast option. Greek yogurt is a great source of protein and probiotics, while fruits and nuts provide fiber, vitamins, and minerals.

Ingredients:

- 1 cup plain Greek yogurt: Greek yogurt is high in protein and low in fat.
- 1/2 cup mixed berries (such as blueberries, strawberries, or raspberries): Berries are rich in antioxidants and beneficial for heart health.
- 1/4 cup granola: Choose a low-sugar, whole grain granola for added crunch and fiber.
- 2 tablespoons chopped nuts (such as almonds, walnuts, or pistachios): Nuts are a good source of heart-healthy fats and provide additional texture and flavor.

- 1 teaspoon honey or maple syrup (optional): Use sparingly as a natural sweetener.

Instructions:

1. In a glass or bowl, layer half of the Greek yogurt.
2. Add half of the mixed berries on top of the yogurt.
3. Sprinkle half of the granola and chopped nuts over the berries.
4. Repeat the layering process with the remaining ingredients.
5. Drizzle honey or maple syrup (if desired) over the top.
6. Serve chilled and enjoy a satisfying and heart-healthy breakfast.

Whole Wheat Banana Pancakes:

These pancakes are made with whole wheat flour and mashed bananas, providing fiber, potassium, and nutrients. They are a heart-healthy twist on a classic breakfast favorite.

Ingredients:

- 1 cup whole wheat flour: Whole wheat flour is higher in fiber compared to refined white flour.
- 1 teaspoon baking powder: Baking powder helps the pancakes rise and become fluffy.
- 1/2 teaspoon cinnamon: Cinnamon adds a warm and comforting flavor while offering potential heart health benefits.
- 1 ripe banana, mashed: Bananas provide natural sweetness and are a good source of potassium.
- 1 cup milk (such as almond milk or low-fat milk): Choose a low-fat or plant-based milk to reduce saturated fat intake.
- 1 large egg: Eggs provide protein and essential nutrients.
- 1 tablespoon honey or maple syrup (optional): Use sparingly, if desired, as a natural sweetener.
- Cooking spray or a small amount of oil for greasing the pan.

Instructions:

1. In a mixing bowl, combine the whole wheat flour, baking powder, and cinnamon.
2. In a separate bowl, whisk together the mashed banana, milk, egg, and honey or maple syrup (if desired).
3. Gradually pour the wet ingredients into the dry ingredients, stirring until just combined. Be careful not to overmix, as it may result in dense pancakes.
4. Heat a non-stick skillet or griddle over medium heat and lightly coat it with cooking spray or a small amount of oil.
5. Pour about 1/4 cup of the pancake batter onto the skillet for each pancake.
6. Cook until bubbles start to form on the surface, then flip and cook the other side until golden brown.
7. Repeat with the remaining batter.
8. Serve the pancakes with a sprinkle of cinnamon, fresh fruit, or a drizzle of honey or maple syrup (if desired).
9. Enjoy a heart-healthy twist on traditional pancakes.

Chapter 2: Low-Sodium Recipes

Lemon Herb Grilled Chicken:

This dish is a heart-healthy option that features lean protein from grilled chicken breasts and incorporates flavorful herbs and spices. By reducing the sodium content in the marinade, it helps individuals manage their blood pressure.

Ingredients:

- 4 boneless, skinless chicken breasts: Skinless chicken breasts are a lean source of protein.
- 2 tablespoons fresh lemon juice: Lemon juice adds a tangy flavor without adding sodium.
- 1 tablespoon olive oil: Olive oil is a healthier fat choice compared to saturated fats.
- 2 cloves garlic, minced: Fresh garlic adds flavor without sodium.
- 1 teaspoon dried thyme: Dried thyme is a sodium-free herb that adds aroma and taste.
- 1 teaspoon dried rosemary: Dried rosemary provides a savory flavor without sodium.

- 1/2 teaspoon black pepper: Black pepper enhances taste without adding sodium.

Instructions:

1. In a small bowl, combine fresh lemon juice, olive oil, minced garlic, dried thyme, dried rosemary, and black pepper.
2. Place the chicken breasts in a shallow dish and pour the marinade over them, ensuring they are evenly coated. Allow them to marinate in the refrigerator for at least 30 minutes.
3. Preheat the grill to medium-high heat.
4. Grill the chicken breasts for about 6-8 minutes per side or until they reach an internal temperature of 165°F (74°C).
5. Remove the chicken from the grill and let it rest for a few minutes before serving.
6. Serve the lemon herb grilled chicken with a side of steamed vegetables and whole grain rice for a flavorful and heart-healthy meal.

Herbed Quinoa Salad:

This salad is a low-sodium dish that combines nutrient-rich ingredients like quinoa, fresh vegetables, and herbs. It provides a good source of fiber, vitamins, and minerals while being flavorful and satisfying.

Ingredients:

- 1 cup cooked quinoa: Quinoa is a whole grain that is naturally low in sodium and high in fiber.
- 1 cup diced cucumbers: Cucumbers add crunch and hydration to the salad without sodium.
- 1 cup halved cherry tomatoes: Cherry tomatoes are a flavorful addition without sodium.
- 1/2 cup chopped fresh parsley: Fresh parsley adds brightness and taste without sodium.
- 1/4 cup chopped fresh mint: Fresh mint enhances flavor without sodium.
- 1/4 cup chopped red onion: Red onion adds a mild onion flavor without sodium.
- 2 tablespoons lemon juice: Lemon juice adds tanginess without sodium.

- 1 tablespoon olive oil: Olive oil provides a healthier fat source compared to high-sodium dressings.
- 1 clove garlic, minced: Fresh garlic adds a savory taste without sodium.
- Salt and pepper to taste: Use minimal amounts of salt, if desired, and incorporate pepper for added flavor.

Instructions:

1. In a large bowl, combine cooked quinoa, diced cucumbers, halved cherry tomatoes, chopped parsley, chopped mint, and chopped red onion.
2. In a small bowl, whisk together lemon juice, olive oil, minced garlic, salt, and pepper.
3. Pour the dressing over the quinoa salad and toss gently to coat all the ingredients.
4. Adjust the seasoning if needed, using minimal amounts of salt.
5. Cover the salad and refrigerate for at least 30 minutes to allow the flavors to meld together.

6. Serve the herbed quinoa salad as a refreshing and low-sodium side dish or as a light main course.

Baked Salmon with Dill and Lemon:

This dish features omega-3 fatty acid-rich salmon, which is known to promote heart health. By using flavorful herbs and lemon instead of high-sodium sauces, it reduces the sodium content while maintaining a delicious taste.

Ingredients:

- 4 salmon fillets: Salmon is an excellent source of heart-healthy omega-3 fatty acids.
- 2 tablespoons fresh dill, chopped: Fresh dill adds a fragrant and savory flavor without sodium.
- 2 tablespoons fresh lemon juice: Lemon juice provides a tangy taste without sodium.
- 1 tablespoon olive oil: Olive oil serves as a healthier alternative to high-sodium oils or butter.

- 2 cloves garlic, minced: Fresh garlic enhances the dish's flavor without adding sodium.
- Salt and pepper to taste: Use minimal amounts of salt, if desired, and incorporate pepper for added taste.

Instructions:

1. Preheat the oven to 375°F (190°C) and lightly grease a baking dish.
2. In a small bowl, mix together chopped dill, lemon juice, olive oil, minced garlic, salt, and pepper.
3. Place the salmon fillets in the prepared baking dish and spoon the dill and lemon mixture over each fillet, ensuring they are evenly coated.
4. Bake the salmon for about 12-15 minutes or until it flakes easily with a fork and reaches an internal temperature of 145°F (63°C).
5. Remove the salmon from the oven and let it rest for a few minutes before serving.
6. Serve the baked salmon with a side of steamed vegetables and a whole grain couscous for a flavorful and heart-healthy meal.

These flavorful dishes with reduced sodium content are not only delicious but also beneficial for individuals looking to manage their blood pressure and reduce the risk of heart disease.

Chapter 3: Plant-Based Meals

Rainbow Veggie Stir-Fry:

This vibrant and nutritious stir-fry incorporates an array of colorful vegetables, providing a variety of vitamins, minerals, and antioxidants. The dish is high in fiber and low in saturated fat, making it heart-healthy.

Ingredients:

- 1 tablespoon olive oil: Olive oil is a healthy fat choice.
- 1 onion, thinly sliced: Onions add flavor and are rich in antioxidants.
- 2 cloves garlic, minced: Garlic enhances taste and has potential heart health benefits.
- 1 red bell pepper, thinly sliced: Red bell peppers are packed with vitamin C and antioxidants.
- 1 yellow bell pepper, thinly sliced: Yellow bell peppers provide additional vitamins and color.

- 1 zucchini, thinly sliced: Zucchini adds a light and refreshing element.
- 1 cup broccoli florets: Broccoli is a cruciferous vegetable that offers heart-protective properties.
- 1 cup snap peas: Snap peas contribute crunch and fiber.
- 1 cup mushrooms, sliced: Mushrooms are low in calories and a good source of minerals.
- 2 tablespoons low-sodium soy sauce: Use a reduced-sodium version to manage sodium intake.
- 1 tablespoon rice vinegar: Rice vinegar adds tanginess without added sodium.
- 1 teaspoon sesame oil: Sesame oil enhances flavor without saturated fat.
- 1 tablespoon sesame seeds: Sesame seeds offer a nutty taste and a source of healthy fats.

Instructions:

1. Heat olive oil in a large skillet or wok over medium-high heat.

2. Add the onion and garlic, and sauté until fragrant and slightly softened.
3. Add the bell peppers, zucchini, broccoli, snap peas, and mushrooms to the skillet. Stir-fry for about 5-7 minutes until the vegetables are crisp-tender.
4. In a small bowl, whisk together the low-sodium soy sauce, rice vinegar, sesame oil, and sesame seeds.
5. Pour the sauce over the stir-fried vegetables and toss to coat evenly.
6. Cook for an additional 1-2 minutes until the sauce thickens slightly.
7. Serve the rainbow veggie stir-fry over cooked brown rice or quinoa for a satisfying and heart-healthy meal.

Lentil and Vegetable Curry:

This hearty and flavorful curry combines protein-rich lentils with an array of vegetables and aromatic spices. It is packed with fiber, vitamins, and minerals, making it an excellent choice for heart health.

Ingredients:

- 1 tablespoon olive oil: Olive oil is a healthier fat option.
- 1 onion, diced: Onions provide flavor and are low in calories.
- 2 cloves garlic, minced: Garlic adds depth of flavor and potential heart health benefits.
- 1 tablespoon grated fresh ginger: Ginger adds a zesty kick and has anti-inflammatory properties.
- 1 tablespoon curry powder: Curry powder infuses the dish with aromatic spices.
- 1 teaspoon ground cumin: Cumin offers a warm and earthy flavor.
- 1 teaspoon ground turmeric: Turmeric adds a vibrant yellow color and potential anti-inflammatory effects.
- 1 cup dried red lentils: Lentils are a great source of plant-based protein and fiber.
- 3 cups vegetable broth: Choose a low-sodium variety to manage sodium intake.
- 1 cup diced tomatoes (fresh or canned): Tomatoes add richness and lycopene, an antioxidant.

- 2 cups chopped mixed vegetables (such as carrots, bell peppers, and cauliflower): Vegetables add texture, nutrients, and color.
- 1 cup coconut milk: Opt for a light version to reduce saturated fat content.
- Fresh cilantro for garnish: Cilantro adds freshness and a pop of flavor.

Instructions:

1. Heat olive oil in a large pot or Dutch oven over medium heat.
2. Add the onion, garlic, and grated ginger, and sauté until fragrant and softened.
3. Stir in the curry powder, cumin, and turmeric, and cook for an additional minute to release the spices' flavors.
4. Add the dried red lentils, vegetable broth, diced tomatoes, and mixed vegetables to the pot. Bring to a boil, then reduce the heat to low, cover, and simmer for about 20-25 minutes, or until the lentils and vegetables are tender.

5. Stir in the coconut milk and simmer for an additional 5 minutes to meld the flavors.
6. Adjust the seasoning if needed.
7. Serve the lentil and vegetable curry over cooked brown rice or whole grain couscous. Garnish with fresh cilantro for added freshness.

Walnut and Berry Oatmeal:

This nutritious and filling oatmeal is packed with heart-healthy ingredients like oats, walnuts, and berries. It provides soluble fiber, omega-3 fatty acids, and antioxidants that support heart health.

Ingredients:

- 1 cup rolled oats: Rolled oats are a great source of soluble fiber.
- 2 cups water or plant-based milk: Choose unsweetened options to reduce added sugars.
- 1/4 cup chopped walnuts: Walnuts provide omega-3 fatty acids and a satisfying crunch.

- 1 cup mixed berries (such as blueberries, strawberries, and raspberries): Berries are rich in antioxidants and natural sweetness.
- 1 tablespoon maple syrup (optional): Add a small amount for natural sweetness.

Instructions:

1. In a saucepan, bring the water or plant-based milk to a boil.
2. Stir in the rolled oats and reduce the heat to medium-low.
3. Cook the oats according to the package instructions, usually for about 5-7 minutes, stirring occasionally until they reach your desired consistency.
4. Remove the saucepan from the heat and stir in the chopped walnuts.
5. Transfer the oatmeal to serving bowls and top with the mixed berries.
6. Drizzle with a small amount of maple syrup if desired for added sweetness.
7. Serve the walnut and berry oatmeal warm for a nourishing and heart-healthy breakfast.

By focusing on fruits, vegetables, whole grains, legumes, and nuts in these plant-based recipes, individuals can benefit from a diet rich in fiber, vitamins, minerals, and antioxidants. This type of diet has been associated with a lower risk of heart disease and improved overall cardiovascular health.

Chapter 4: Lean Protein Options

Grilled Lemon Herb Chicken with Roasted Vegetables:

This recipe features lean chicken breasts and pairs them with a colorful array of roasted vegetables. It's a nutritious and satisfying dish that is easy to prepare.

Ingredients:

- 4 boneless, skinless chicken breasts: Chicken breasts are a lean source of protein.
- 2 tablespoons fresh lemon juice: Lemon juice adds a tangy flavor without adding fat.
- 2 tablespoons olive oil: Olive oil provides healthy fats.
- 2 cloves garlic, minced: Garlic enhances the taste without adding extra calories.
- 1 teaspoon dried thyme: Dried thyme adds a savory flavor without added fat.
- 1 teaspoon dried rosemary: Dried rosemary provides aromatic notes without added fat.

- Salt and pepper to taste: Use minimal amounts of salt, if desired, and incorporate pepper for added flavor.
- 2 cups mixed vegetables (such as bell peppers, zucchini, and cherry tomatoes): Vegetables add fiber and nutrients.

Instructions:

1. In a bowl, whisk together the fresh lemon juice, olive oil, minced garlic, dried thyme, dried rosemary, salt, and pepper.
2. Place the chicken breasts in a shallow dish and pour the marinade over them, ensuring they are evenly coated. Let them marinate in the refrigerator for at least 30 minutes.
3. Preheat the grill to medium-high heat.
4. Grill the chicken breasts for about 6-8 minutes per side or until they reach an internal temperature of 165°F (74°C).
5. While the chicken is grilling, preheat the oven to 425°F (220°C) and prepare a baking sheet.

6. Toss the mixed vegetables with a drizzle of olive oil, salt, and pepper. Spread them out on the baking sheet.

7. Roast the vegetables for about 15-20 minutes or until they are tender and slightly charred.

8. Serve the grilled lemon herb chicken alongside the roasted vegetables for a protein-packed and flavorful meal.

Baked Salmon with Quinoa and Spinach Salad:

This recipe combines heart-healthy salmon with a nutritious quinoa and spinach salad. It's a well-balanced meal that is rich in omega-3 fatty acids, protein, and fiber.

Ingredients:

- 4 salmon fillets: Salmon is a great source of omega-3 fatty acids.
- 2 tablespoons olive oil: Olive oil provides healthy fats.
- 2 teaspoons Dijon mustard: Dijon mustard adds tanginess without adding many calories.

- 2 cloves garlic, minced: Garlic enhances the taste without adding extra calories.
- 1 teaspoon dried dill: Dried dill provides a refreshing flavor without added fat.
- Salt and pepper to taste: Use minimal amounts of salt, if desired, and incorporate pepper for added flavor.
- 1 cup cooked quinoa: Quinoa is a protein-rich whole grain.
- 2 cups fresh spinach leaves: Spinach adds fiber and nutrients.

Instructions:

1. Preheat the oven to 375°F (190°C) and lightly grease a baking dish.
2. In a small bowl, whisk together the olive oil, Dijon mustard, minced garlic, dried dill, salt, and pepper.
3. Place the salmon fillets in the prepared baking dish and brush the mustard mixture over each fillet, ensuring they are evenly coated.

4. Bake the salmon for about 12-15 minutes or until it flakes easily with a fork and reaches an internal temperature of 145°F (63°C).

5. While the salmon is baking, prepare the quinoa according to the package instructions.

6. In a large bowl, combine the cooked quinoa and fresh spinach leaves. Toss well to wilt the spinach slightly.

7. Season the quinoa and spinach salad with salt, pepper, and a drizzle of olive oil if desired.

8. Serve the baked salmon over a bed of the quinoa and spinach salad for a nutritious and satisfying meal.

Tofu and Vegetable Stir-Fry:

This recipe features protein-packed tofu and an assortment of colorful vegetables, creating a flavorful and nutrient-rich stir-fry.

Ingredients:

- 14 oz (400g) firm tofu, drained and cut into cubes: Tofu is a versatile plant-based protein source.

- 2 tablespoons soy sauce: Use a reduced-sodium version to manage sodium intake.
- 1 tablespoon hoisin sauce: Hoisin sauce adds a rich and savory taste.
- 1 tablespoon rice vinegar: Rice vinegar provides a tangy flavor without added fat.
- 1 tablespoon cornstarch: Cornstarch helps thicken the sauce.
- 1 tablespoon vegetable oil: Vegetable oil is used for stir-frying.
- 1 onion, thinly sliced: Onions add flavor and are low in calories.
- 2 bell peppers, thinly sliced: Bell peppers provide crunch and additional nutrients.
- 2 cups broccoli florets: Broccoli is a cruciferous vegetable that offers health benefits.
- 1 cup snap peas: Snap peas contribute texture and fiber.
- 2 cloves garlic, minced: Garlic enhances the taste without adding extra calories.
- Sesame seeds for garnish (optional): Sesame seeds add a nutty flavor and visual appeal.

Instructions:

1. In a small bowl, whisk together the soy sauce, hoisin sauce, rice vinegar, and cornstarch. Set aside.
2. Heat vegetable oil in a large skillet or wok over medium-high heat.
3. Add the onion, bell peppers, broccoli, snap peas, and minced garlic to the skillet. Stir-fry for about 5-7 minutes until the vegetables are crisp-tender.
4. Push the vegetables to one side of the skillet and add the tofu cubes to the empty space. Cook for a few minutes until the tofu is heated through.
5. Give the sauce mixture a stir and pour it over the tofu and vegetables. Stir-fry for an additional minute or until the sauce thickens and coats everything evenly.
6. Remove from heat and sprinkle with sesame seeds, if desired, for garnish.
7. Serve the tofu and vegetable stir-fry over cooked brown rice or whole wheat noodles for a protein-rich and satisfying meal.

By incorporating lean protein sources like skinless poultry, fish, tofu, or legumes into these recipes, individuals can enjoy flavorful and nutritious meals that support heart health.

Chapter 5: Heart-Healthy Snacks

Homemade Granola Bars:

These homemade granola bars are packed with wholesome ingredients like oats, nuts, seeds, and dried fruits. They are a delicious and convenient snack option that provides fiber, healthy fats, and antioxidants.

Ingredients:

- 1 ½ cups rolled oats: Rolled oats are a great source of fiber.
- ½ cup chopped nuts (such as almonds, walnuts, or cashews): Nuts provide healthy fats and protein.
- ¼ cup honey or maple syrup: Use a natural sweetener for a touch of sweetness.
- ¼ cup nut butter (such as almond butter or peanut butter): Nut butter adds richness and binds the ingredients together.
- 2 tablespoons ground flaxseed: Flaxseed is a source of omega-3 fatty acids and fiber.

- 2 tablespoons dried fruit (such as cranberries, raisins, or chopped dates): Dried fruit adds natural sweetness and texture.
- 1 teaspoon vanilla extract: Vanilla extract enhances the flavor.
- ¼ teaspoon salt: Use a small amount of salt to enhance the taste.

Instructions:

1. Preheat the oven to 350°F (175°C) and line a baking dish with parchment paper.
2. In a large mixing bowl, combine the rolled oats, chopped nuts, ground flaxseed, and dried fruit.
3. In a small saucepan, warm the honey or maple syrup and nut butter over low heat until they are melted and well combined.
4. Remove the saucepan from heat and stir in the vanilla extract and salt.
5. Pour the wet ingredients over the dry ingredients and mix until everything is evenly coated.

6. Transfer the mixture to the lined baking dish and press it down firmly to create an even layer.
7. Bake for about 15-20 minutes or until the edges turn golden brown.
8. Allow the granola bars to cool completely before cutting them into bars or squares.
9. Store the homemade granola bars in an airtight container for up to one week.

Fruit Skewers with Yogurt Dip:

These fruit skewers with yogurt dip are a refreshing and nutritious snack that combines the natural sweetness of fruits with a protein-rich dip. They are packed with vitamins, minerals, and antioxidants.

Ingredients:

- Assorted fresh fruits (such as strawberries, grapes, pineapple chunks, and melon balls): Fruits provide natural sugars and various nutrients.
- Wooden skewers: Skewers are used for assembling the fruit kebabs.

- 1 cup plain Greek yogurt: Greek yogurt is a good source of protein.
- 1 tablespoon honey: Honey adds a touch of sweetness, if desired.
- ½ teaspoon vanilla extract: Vanilla extract enhances the flavor.

Instructions:

1. Wash and prepare the fresh fruits by cutting them into bite-sized pieces.
2. Thread the fruit pieces onto the wooden skewers, alternating between different fruits to create colorful combinations.
3. In a small bowl, whisk together the plain Greek yogurt, honey, and vanilla extract until well combined.
4. Serve the fruit skewers with the yogurt dip on the side for dipping.
5. Enjoy the refreshing combination of fruits and yogurt dip as a healthy and satisfying snack.

Roasted Chickpeas:

Roasted chickpeas are a crunchy and protein-packed snack that can be customized with various seasonings. They are a great alternative to processed snacks and provide fiber, vitamins, and minerals.

Ingredients:

- 1 can chickpeas (15 ounces), drained and rinsed: Chickpeas are a good source of protein and fiber.
- 1 tablespoon olive oil: Olive oil adds a light coating and healthy fats.
- Seasonings of your choice (such as paprika, cumin, chili powder, or garlic powder): Choose your preferred seasonings for added flavor.
- Salt to taste: Use a small amount of salt to enhance the taste.

Instructions:

1. Preheat the oven to 400°F (200°C) and line a baking sheet with parchment paper.

2. Place the drained and rinsed chickpeas on the baking sheet and pat them dry with a paper towel.
3. Drizzle the chickpeas with olive oil and toss them to ensure they are coated evenly.
4. Sprinkle your desired seasonings and salt over the chickpeas, and toss them again to distribute the seasonings.
5. Spread the chickpeas out in a single layer on the baking sheet.
6. Roast the chickpeas in the preheated oven for about 25-30 minutes or until they become crispy and golden brown.
7. Remove the chickpeas from the oven and let them cool before enjoying.
8. Store the roasted chickpeas in an airtight container for up to one week.

These satisfying and heart-healthy snacks offer a range of flavors and textures while providing essential nutrients.

Chapter 6: Mediterranean-Inspired Recipes

The Mediterranean diet is known for its heart-protective benefits, incorporating olive oil, whole grains, fresh fruits and vegetables, and moderate amounts of lean proteins. Here are four recipes that showcase the Mediterranean diet:

Greek Salad:

This refreshing and nutritious salad combines crisp vegetables, tangy feta cheese, and a simple dressing made with olive oil and lemon juice. It's a light and flavorful dish that is packed with antioxidants and healthy fats.

Ingredients:

- 2 medium cucumbers, diced: Cucumbers add crunch and hydration.
- 2 cups cherry tomatoes, halved: Cherry tomatoes provide a burst of sweetness.

- 1 medium red onion, thinly sliced: Red onions add a mild pungent flavor.
- 1 green bell pepper, diced: Bell peppers contribute a vibrant color and crunch.
- 1 cup Kalamata olives, pitted: Kalamata olives offer a rich and savory taste.
- 4 ounces feta cheese, crumbled: Feta cheese provides a creamy and tangy element.
- 2 tablespoons extra-virgin olive oil: Olive oil is a key component of the Mediterranean diet.
- 1 tablespoon freshly squeezed lemon juice: Lemon juice adds a bright and tangy flavor.
- 1 teaspoon dried oregano: Dried oregano adds an earthy and herbal note.
- Salt and pepper to taste: Use a minimal amount of salt and pepper, if desired.

Instructions:

1. In a large salad bowl, combine the diced cucumbers, halved cherry tomatoes, sliced red onion, diced green bell pepper, and pitted Kalamata olives.

2. In a small bowl, whisk together the extra-virgin olive oil, lemon juice, dried oregano, salt, and pepper.
3. Drizzle the dressing over the salad ingredients and toss gently to combine.
4. Add the crumbled feta cheese on top of the salad.
5. Serve the Greek salad chilled as a refreshing and nutritious side dish or a light meal.

Roasted Mediterranean Vegetables with Whole Wheat Couscous:

This vibrant and flavorful dish features a medley of roasted vegetables seasoned with Mediterranean herbs, served over whole wheat couscous. It's a wholesome and satisfying meal that showcases the abundance of fresh produce in the Mediterranean region.

Ingredients:

- 1 eggplant, diced: Eggplant adds a creamy texture and rich flavor.
- 2 zucchini, diced: Zucchini contributes a mild and tender element.
- 1 red bell pepper, sliced: Red bell peppers provide a sweet and vibrant taste.
- 1 yellow bell pepper, sliced: Yellow bell peppers add a slightly milder flavor and bright color.
- 1 red onion, sliced: Red onions add a sweet and tangy note.
- 2 tablespoons extra-virgin olive oil: Olive oil enhances the flavors and promotes heart health.
- 1 teaspoon dried oregano: Dried oregano adds a savory and earthy taste.
- 1 teaspoon dried basil: Dried basil provides a fragrant and herbal flavor.
- Salt and pepper to taste: Use a minimal amount of salt and pepper, if desired.
- 1 cup whole wheat couscous: Whole wheat couscous is a nutritious whole grain option.

- Fresh parsley for garnish (optional): Fresh parsley adds a pop of freshness and color.

Instructions:

1. Preheat the oven to 425°F (220°C) and line a baking sheet with parchment paper.
2. In a large bowl, combine the diced eggplant, diced zucchini, sliced red and yellow bell peppers, and sliced red onion.
3. Drizzle the extra-virgin olive oil over the vegetables and sprinkle with dried oreg

Baked Lemon Herb Salmon:

Salmon is a rich source of omega-3 fatty acids, which are known to promote heart health. This recipe combines the flavors of fresh herbs and zesty lemon to create a delicious and nutritious dish.

Ingredients:

- 4 salmon fillets (4-6 ounces each): Salmon is a lean source of protein and heart-healthy omega-3 fatty acids.
- 2 tablespoons extra-virgin olive oil: Olive oil adds richness and promotes heart health.
- 2 tablespoons freshly squeezed lemon juice: Lemon juice provides a bright and tangy flavor.
- 2 cloves garlic, minced: Garlic enhances the taste without adding extra calories.
- 1 teaspoon dried dill: Dried dill adds a refreshing and herbal note.
- 1 teaspoon dried thyme: Dried thyme adds depth of flavor.
- Salt and pepper to taste: Use a minimal amount of salt and pepper, if desired.
- Lemon slices for garnish (optional): Lemon slices add visual appeal.

Instructions:

1. Preheat the oven to 375°F (190°C) and line a baking sheet with parchment paper.
2. In a small bowl, whisk together the extra-virgin olive oil, lemon juice, minced garlic, dried dill, dried thyme, salt, and pepper.
3. Place the salmon fillets on the prepared baking sheet.
4. Drizzle the lemon herb mixture over the salmon fillets, ensuring they are evenly coated.
5. Bake in the preheated oven for about 12-15 minutes, or until the salmon is cooked through and flakes easily with a fork.
6. Remove from the oven and let the salmon rest for a few minutes.
7. Garnish with lemon slices, if desired, and serve the baked lemon herb salmon with a side of roasted vegetables or whole grains for a complete and heart-healthy meal.

Quinoa Stuffed Bell Peppers:

This colorful and flavorful dish features bell peppers stuffed with a filling of quinoa, vegetables, and herbs.

It's a nutritious and satisfying option that showcases the versatility of quinoa and the abundance of vegetables in the Mediterranean diet.

Ingredients:

- 4 bell peppers (assorted colors): Bell peppers provide a vibrant and sweet taste.
- 1 cup cooked quinoa: Quinoa is a protein-rich whole grain.
- 1 small onion, finely chopped: Onion adds flavor and is low in calories.
- 2 cloves garlic, minced: Garlic enhances the taste without adding extra calories.
- 1 medium zucchini, diced: Zucchini adds a tender and mild element.
- 1 medium tomato, diced: Tomato adds juiciness and a touch of sweetness.
- 1 cup baby spinach leaves: Spinach provides a nutritional boost.
- ¼ cup chopped fresh parsley: Fresh parsley adds freshness and flavor.

- 2 tablespoons extra-virgin olive oil: Olive oil enhances the flavors and promotes heart health.
- 1 teaspoon dried oregano: Dried oregano adds a savory and earthy taste.
- Salt and pepper to taste: Use a minimal amount of salt and pepper, if desired.

Instructions:

1. Preheat the oven to 375°F (190°C) and line a baking dish with parchment paper.
2. Slice off the tops of the bell peppers and remove the seeds and membranes. Set the hollowed bell peppers aside.
3. In a large skillet, heat the extra-virgin olive oil over medium heat.
4. Add the chopped onion and minced garlic to the skillet and sauté until they become translucent and fragrant.
5. Stir in the diced zucchini, diced tomato, and baby spinach leaves. Cook for a few minutes until the vegetables are tender.

6. Remove the skillet from the heat and add the cooked quinoa, chopped fresh parsley, dried oregano, salt, and pepper. Mix well to combine all the ingredients.
7. Stuff the hollowed bell peppers with the quinoa and vegetable mixture and place them in the prepared baking dish.
8. Cover the dish with aluminum foil and bake in the preheated oven for about 25-30 minutes, or until the bell peppers are tender and the filling is heated through.
9. Remove from the oven and let the stuffed bell peppers cool slightly before serving.
10. Serve the quinoa stuffed bell peppers as a wholesome and flavorful main dish, accompanied by a side salad or a serving of roasted Mediterranean vegetables.

These recipes showcase the heart-protective benefits of the Mediterranean diet by incorporating wholesome ingredients and flavorful combinations. Enjoy these dishes as part of a well-balanced and heart-healthy meal plan.

Chapter 7: Desserts with a Heart-Healthy Twist

Fruit Salad with Honey-Lime Dressing:

This refreshing and naturally sweet fruit salad is a perfect choice for a healthier dessert option. The honey-lime dressing adds a hint of sweetness without excessive added sugars.

Ingredients:

- Assorted fresh fruits (such as berries, melon, grapes, and citrus segments): Use a variety of colorful fruits for a vibrant and flavorful salad.
- 1 tablespoon honey: Honey provides a natural sweetness.
- 1 tablespoon freshly squeezed lime juice: Lime juice adds a tangy flavor.
- Fresh mint leaves for garnish (optional): Mint leaves add freshness and visual appeal.

Instructions:

1. Wash and prepare the fresh fruits by cutting them into bite-sized pieces.
2. In a small bowl, whisk together the honey and lime juice until well combined.
3. Place the prepared fruits in a serving bowl and drizzle the honey-lime dressing over them.
4. Gently toss the fruit salad to coat the fruits with the dressing.
5. Garnish with fresh mint leaves, if desired.
6. Serve the fruit salad immediately for a light and naturally sweet dessert.

Yogurt Parfait:

Yogurt parfaits are a nutritious and satisfying dessert option. They combine creamy yogurt, layers of fresh fruits, and a crunchy topping for added texture and flavor.

Ingredients:

- 1 cup Greek yogurt: Greek yogurt provides a creamy and protein-rich base.
- Assorted fresh fruits (such as berries, sliced bananas, or diced mango): Choose your favorite fruits for layering.
- 2 tablespoons granola: Granola adds crunch and a hint of sweetness.
- 1 tablespoon honey or maple syrup (optional): Use a small amount of sweetener, if desired.

Instructions:

1. In a glass or serving dish, start by layering a spoonful of Greek yogurt at the bottom.
2. Add a layer of fresh fruits on top of the yogurt.
3. Repeat the layers of yogurt and fruits until the glass or dish is filled.
4. Sprinkle granola on the final layer for a crunchy topping.
5. Drizzle honey or maple syrup over the parfait for added sweetness, if desired.
6. Serve the yogurt parfait immediately or refrigerate until ready to enjoy.

Dark Chocolate-Dipped Berries:

Dark chocolate is a healthier alternative to milk chocolate, as it contains higher amounts of cocoa solids and lower levels of added sugars. Pair it with antioxidant-rich berries for a delicious and guilt-free dessert.

Ingredients:

- Assorted fresh berries (such as strawberries, raspberries, or blueberries): Choose your favorite berries for dipping.
- 2 ounces dark chocolate (70% cocoa or higher), chopped: Dark chocolate with higher cocoa content is recommended for its health benefits.

Instructions:

1. Wash and dry the fresh berries thoroughly.
2. In a microwave-safe bowl, melt the dark chocolate in the microwave in short intervals, stirring in between, until smooth and melted.

3. Holding each berry by its stem or using a toothpick, dip it into the melted dark chocolate, coating about two-thirds of the berry.
4. Place the dipped berries on a parchment-lined baking sheet.
5. Repeat the process with the remaining berries.
6. Place the baking sheet with the dipped berries in the refrigerator for about 15-20 minutes, or until the chocolate sets.
7. Once the chocolate is firm, remove the berries from the refrigerator and serve them as a delightful and healthier chocolate treat.

These desserts offer alternatives to traditional sugary and high-fat options, allowing you to satisfy your sweet tooth while making healthier choices. Enjoy these delicious treats as part of a well-balanced diet.

Chapter 8: Cooking Techniques for Heart Health

Tips and techniques for reducing the use of unhealthy fats and incorporating healthier cooking methods:

Replace Unhealthy Fats:

- Choose healthier fats: Opt for healthier fats like olive oil, avocado oil, or coconut oil instead of butter or lard. These oils are rich in monounsaturated fats or medium-chain triglycerides (MCTs) that can be beneficial for heart health.
- Use non-stick cookware: Utilize non-stick pans or cooking sprays to reduce the need for excessive amounts of cooking oil.

Healthy Cooking Methods:

- Grilling: Grilling is a great way to add flavor to foods without the need for excessive fats. Grill lean proteins like skinless chicken breast, fish fillets, or vegetables for a delicious and healthy meal.

- Baking: Baking is a low-fat cooking method that can create flavorful and tender dishes. Try baking fish, chicken, or vegetables with a drizzle of olive oil and a sprinkle of herbs and spices for added taste.
- Steaming: Steaming is a gentle and fat-free cooking method that helps retain the natural flavors and nutrients of foods. Steam vegetables, seafood, or poultry to maintain their tenderness and enhance their natural taste.
- Roasting: Roasting allows foods to caramelize and develop a rich flavor without excessive added fats. Roast vegetables, chicken, or tofu with a light coating of olive oil and your favorite herbs and spices.

Flavor Enhancers:

- Herbs and spices: Use a variety of herbs and spices to add flavor to your dishes without relying on unhealthy fats. Experiment with garlic, ginger, turmeric, cumin, paprika, or rosemary to enhance the taste of your meals.

- Citrus juices and zest: Fresh citrus juices, such as lemon or lime, can add brightness to your dishes. Additionally, using the zest of citrus fruits can provide a burst of flavor without adding fats.
- Vinegars: Add depth and tang to your dishes with different types of vinegars, such as balsamic vinegar, apple cider vinegar, or rice vinegar. They can be used to create flavorful dressings, marinades, or sauces.

Portion Control:

- Keep an eye on portion sizes: Even with healthier cooking methods and ingredients, it's important to practice portion control to maintain a balanced diet. Be mindful of the amount of food you consume to avoid overeating.

Preparation Techniques:

- Trim visible fat: Trim any visible fat from meats before cooking to reduce the overall fat content.
- Use leaner cuts of meat: Opt for lean cuts of meat, such as skinless poultry, lean beef, or pork loin, to reduce the saturated fat content in your meals.
- Remove skin from poultry: Poultry skin contains a significant amount of saturated fat. Removing the skin before cooking can make your dish healthier.
- Drain excess fats: When cooking ground meats, drain off excess fat after browning to reduce the fat content in your dish.

By incorporating these tips and techniques into your cooking routine, you can reduce the use of unhealthy fats while embracing healthier cooking methods and still enjoy flavorful and nutritious meals.

Chapter 9: Ingredient Substitutions

Educational segment about healthier alternatives to common ingredients, along with recipe ideas that showcase these substitutions:

Healthier Alternatives for Fats and Oils:

Replace butter with unsaturated oils: Swap out butter, which is high in saturated fat, with healthier options like olive oil, avocado oil, or canola oil. These unsaturated oils are rich in monounsaturated or polyunsaturated fats, which can be beneficial for heart health.

- Recipe idea: Mediterranean Quinoa Salad
- In a large bowl, combine cooked quinoa, diced cucumbers, cherry tomatoes, chopped fresh parsley, and crumbled feta cheese.
- In a separate small bowl, whisk together extra-virgin olive oil, freshly squeezed lemon juice, minced garlic, dried oregano, salt, and pepper to make the dressing.

- Drizzle the dressing over the quinoa salad and toss gently to combine. Serve chilled.

Healthier Alternatives for Flours:

Use whole wheat flour instead of refined flour: Whole wheat flour is a healthier choice as it retains the fiber and nutrients found in the whole grain. Substitute whole wheat flour for refined flour in baking recipes like bread, muffins, or pancakes.

- Recipe idea: Whole Wheat Banana Bread
- In a mixing bowl, mash ripe bananas and add melted coconut oil, honey, Greek yogurt, eggs, and vanilla extract. Mix well.
- In a separate bowl, combine whole wheat flour, baking soda, cinnamon, and a pinch of salt.
- Gradually add the dry ingredients to the wet ingredients and mix until just combined.
- Pour the batter into a greased loaf pan and bake in a preheated oven at 350°F (175°C) for about 50-60 minutes or until a toothpick inserted into the center comes out clean. Allow it to cool before slicing.

Healthier Alternatives for Sweeteners:

Choose natural sweeteners over refined sugars: Instead of using refined white sugar, opt for natural sweeteners like honey, maple syrup, or dates. These options provide sweetness along with additional nutrients.

- Recipe idea: Oatmeal Raisin Energy Bites
- In a food processor, combine rolled oats, almond butter, honey, vanilla extract, ground cinnamon, and a pinch of salt. Process until well combined.
- Add raisins and pulse a few times to incorporate them into the mixture.
- Roll the mixture into small bite-sized balls and refrigerate for about 30 minutes to firm up before serving.

Healthier Alternatives for Dairy Products:

Use Greek yogurt instead of sour cream or mayonnaise: Greek yogurt is a healthier substitute for sour cream or mayonnaise in recipes. It provides creaminess and tang while being lower in fat and higher in protein.

- Recipe idea: Greek Yogurt Ranch Dip
- In a bowl, mix together Greek yogurt, dried dill, garlic powder, onion powder, dried parsley, lemon juice, salt, and pepper.
- Stir well until all the ingredients are combined. Adjust the seasoning according to taste.
- Cover the dip and refrigerate for at least 30 minutes to allow the flavors to meld. Serve with vegetable sticks or whole grain crackers.

By incorporating these healthier alternatives into your cooking and baking, you can enhance the nutritional value of your meals while still enjoying delicious flavors. Experiment with these substitutions and adapt them to your favorite recipes to make them more wholesome and nutritious.

Chapter 10: Meal Planning and Portion Control

Guidance on planning heart-healthy meals and portion control tips to help individuals maintain a balanced diet and manage their calorie intake effectively:

Planning Heart-Healthy Meals:

- Include a variety of fruits and vegetables: Aim to incorporate a colorful assortment of fruits and vegetables into your meals. These are rich in vitamins, minerals, and fiber that promote heart health.
- Choose whole grains: Opt for whole grain products like whole wheat bread, brown rice, and whole grain pasta. These contain more fiber and nutrients compared to refined grains.
- Include lean proteins: Include lean protein sources such as skinless poultry, fish, legumes, tofu, or tempeh. These provide essential nutrients without excessive saturated fats.

- Limit sodium intake: Use herbs, spices, and other flavor enhancers to season your meals instead of relying on excessive salt. This helps reduce the risk of high blood pressure.
- Incorporate healthy fats: Include sources of healthy fats like avocados, nuts, seeds, and olive oil. These can benefit heart health when consumed in moderation.

Portion Control Tips:

- Use smaller plates and bowls: Serving your meals on smaller plates and bowls can create the illusion of a fuller plate and help control portion sizes.
- Fill half your plate with vegetables: Make vegetables the star of your meals by filling half of your plate with non-starchy vegetables like leafy greens, broccoli, peppers, or cauliflower.
- Measure portions: Use measuring cups, spoons, or a food scale to accurately measure portion sizes, especially for calorie-dense foods like nuts, seeds, or grains.

- Be mindful of condiments and dressings: Pay attention to the amount of salad dressings, sauces, and condiments you use, as they can add significant calories. Opt for lighter options or use them sparingly.
- Listen to your body's hunger and fullness cues: Eat slowly and pay attention to your body's signals of hunger and fullness. Stop eating when you feel satisfied, not overly full.
- Be aware of high-calorie beverages: Many beverages, including soda, fruit juices, and sweetened drinks, can be high in calories. Choose water, herbal tea, or unsweetened beverages as your primary choices.

Balanced Meal Examples:

- Grilled chicken breast with a side of roasted vegetables and quinoa.
- Baked salmon served with steamed broccoli and a quinoa salad.
- Stir-fried tofu with mixed vegetables and brown rice.

- Spinach salad topped with grilled shrimp, cherry tomatoes, and a light vinaigrette dressing.
- Lentil soup with a side of whole grain bread and a mixed green salad.

Remember, portion control is essential for maintaining a balanced diet and managing calorie intake.

It's good to have you here. I hope you found this guide helpful?

Now this is your special gift: Email me on duncanhealthcare01@gmail.com to get a free ebook on keto diet cookbook

Happy Cooking!

www.ingramcontent.com/pod-product-compliance
Lightning Source LLC
Chambersburg PA
CBHW072339270726

48659CB00022B/2012